47 Colon Cancer Juice Recipes:

Quickly and Naturally Feed Your Body the Nutrients it needs to Boost Your Immune System and Fight Cancer Cells

By

Joe Correa CSN

COPYRIGHT

ACKNOWLEDGEMENTS

This book is dedicated to my friends and family that have had mild or serious illnesses so that you may find a solution and make the necessary changes in your life.

47 Colon Cancer Juice Recipes:

Quickly and Naturally Feed Your Body the Nutrients it needs to Boost Your Immune System and Fight Cancer Cells

By

Joe Correa CSN

CONTENTS

ABOUT THE AUTHOR

After years of Research, I honestly believe in the positive effects that proper nutrition can have over the body and mind. My knowledge and experience has helped me live healthier throughout the years and which I have shared with family and friends. The more you know about eating and drinking healthier, the sooner you will want to change your life and eating habits.

Nutrition is a key part in the process of being healthy and living longer so get started today. The first step is the most important and the most significant.

INTRODUCTION

47 Colon Cancer Juice Recipes: Quickly and Naturally Feed Your Body the Nutrients it needs to Boost Your Immune System and Fight Cancer Cells

By Joe Correa CSN

Colon cancer is a common disease which happens when tumorous growths develop in the large intestine. This serious disease is the third most common cause of cancer-related deaths in the United States which is why recognizing the symptoms and changing some lifestyle habits can be a lifesaver.

The most common symptoms you definitely have to keep in check are:

- A sudden change in your bowel movements
- Any type of rectal bleeding is a potential colon cancer symptom
- Intense abdominal pain
- Frequent weakness or fatigue
- Sudden and unexplained weight loss

However, you have to keep in mind that most people don't experience any of these symptoms in the early stages of the disease. This is why a regular physical exam is very important if for some reason you suspect abnormalities.

Another important step you have to take in order to prevent this terrible and extremely dangerous disease is definitely a dietary lifestyle change. This life-saving decision will permanently change the way you eat, and most importantly, a healthy diet will change the way your digestive tract handles food. This means that with just a couple of simple steps, your body will start to change and you will feel much better. You will have to change the way you eat and adopt some long-term diet habits. Only this will permanently clean your digestive tract and reduce the risk of colon cancer.

But, I have to point out that in order to be 100% sure you're healthy, the diet, by itself, won't be enough. A healthy diet combined with regular exercise is the only way to successfully fight off this disease.

This beautiful collection of colon cancer preventing juice recipes will become your guide in leading a healthy life. These juices are full of fibers that will clean your entire digestive tract and wash away all the toxins you've been collecting over the years. But, that's not all, these juices were carefully chosen to fully satisfy your taste and make you want more! They are amazingly simple to prepare.

Within just a couple of minutes you will have a glass full of nutrients your body needs on a daily basis.

Make sure to try them all and I wish you the best luck in your journey back to health!

47 COLON CANCER JUICE RECIPES: QUICKLY AND NATURALLY FEED YOUR BODY THE NUTRIENTS IT NEEDS TO BOOST YOUR IMMUNE SYSTEM AND FIGHT CANCER CELLS

1.   Apple Ginger Juice

Ingredients:

1 large Granny Smith's apple, cored

½ cup of collard greens

1 tsp of ginger, ground

1 large cucumber

¼ cup of fresh parsley

Preparation:

Wash the apple and cut lengthwise in half. Remove the core and chop into small pieces. Set aside.

Wash the collard greens thoroughly under cold running water using a large colander. Drain and torn into small pieces. Set aside.

Wash the cucumber and cut into thin slices. Set aside.

Rinse the parsley and chop into small pieces. Set aside.

Now, combine apple, collard greens, cucumber, and parsley in a juicer and process until juiced. trans

Transfer to serving glasses and add few ice cubes.

Serve immediately.

Nutritional information per serving: Kcal: 96, Protein: 3.1g, Carbs: 28.7g, Fats: 1.2g

2.   Carrot Turnip Juice

Ingredients:

2 large carrots, sliced

1 cup of turnip greens, torn

1 cup of cauliflower, chopped

1 large radish, chopped

¼ tsp of ginger, ground

2 oz of water

Preparation:

Wash and peel the carrots. Cut into thin slices and set aside.

Wash the turnip greens thoroughly under cold running water. Drain and torn into small pieces. Set aside.

Trim off the outer leaves of the cauliflower. Wash it and chop into small pieces. Fill the measuring cup and reserve the rest for later.

Wash the radish and chop into small pieces. Set aside.

Wash the radish and chop into small pieces. Set aside.

Now, combine cauliflower, carrots, radish, and turnip greens in a juicer and process until juiced. Transfer to a serving glass and stir in the ginger and water.

Add some ice and serve immediately.

Nutritional information per serving: Kcal: 75, Protein: 4.3g, Carbs: 23.3g, Fats: 0.8g

3.   Lemon Grapefruit Juice

Ingredients:

2 whole lemons, peeled and halved

1 whole grapefruit, peeled and wedged

1 cup of mango, chunked

1 small Granny Smith's apple, cored

¼ tsp of ginger, ground

Preparation:

Peel the lemons and cut each lengthwise in half. Set aside.

Peel the grapefruit and divide into wedges. Cut each wedge in half and set aside.

Peel the mango and cut into chunks. Fill the measuring cup and reserve the rest for later. Set aside.

Wash the apple and cut lengthwise in half. Remove the core and cut into bite-sized pieces. Set aside.

Now, combine lemon, mango, grapefruit, and apple in a juicer and process until juiced. Transfer to a serving glass and stir in the ginger.

Add few ice cubes and serve immediately.

Enjoy!

Nutritional information per serving: Kcal: 65, Protein: 4.5g, Carbs: 16.8g, Fats: 0.8g

4.   Apple Celery Juice

Ingredients:

1 small Golden Delicious apple, cored

1 cup of celery, chopped

1 cup of apricots, chopped

1 cup of strawberries, chopped

¼ tsp of cinnamon, ground

Preparation:

Wash the apple and cut lengthwise in half. Remove the core and cut into small pieces. Set aside.

Wash the celery and chop into small pieces. Set aside.

Wash the apricots and cut in half. Remove the pits and chop into small pieces. Fill the measuring cup and reserve the rest for later. Set aside.

Wash the strawberries and remove the stems. Cut into small pieces and fill the measuring cup. Reserve the rest for later.

Now, combine apple,celery, apricots, and strawberries in a juicer and process until juiced. Transfer to a serving glass and stir in the cinnamon.

Add some ice and serve immediately.

Nutritional information per serving: Kcal: 170, Protein: 4.3g, Carbs: 49.9g, Fats: 1.4g

5.   Broccoli Lime Juice

Ingredients:

2 cups of broccoli, chopped

1 whole lime, peeled and halved

2 cups of kale, chopped

1 cup of cucumber, sliced

1 whole lemon, peeled and halved

1 oz of water

Preparation:

Wash the broccoli and trim off the outer leaves. Cut into small pieces and fill the measuring cup. Reserve the rest in the refrigerator.

Peel the lime and lemon. Cut each fruit lengthwise in half and set aside.

Wash the kale thoroughly under cold running water. Drain and chop into small pieces. Set aside.

Wash the cucumber and cut into thin slices. Fill the measuring cup and reserve the rest for later.

Now, combine broccoli, kale, cucumber, lime, and lemon in a juicer and process until juiced. Transfer to a serving glass and stir in the water.

Sprinkle with some mint for some extra taste, but it's optional.

Refrigerate for 10 minutes before serving.

Enjoy!

Nutritional information per serving: Kcal: 116, Protein: 12.1g, Carbs: 34.8g, Fats: 2.2g

6.   Lemon Pineapple Juice

Ingredients:

1 whole lemon, peeled

1 cup of black grapes

1 cup of pineapple, chunked

1 whole grapefruit, peeled and wedged

¼ tsp of cinnamon, ground

Preparation:

Peel the lemon and cut lengthwise in half. Set aside.

Using a sharp paring knife, cut the top of the pineapple. Gently remove all hard skin and cut into chunks. Fill the measuring cup and reserve the in the refrigerator.

Rinse the grapes thoroughly under cold running water. Remove the stems and fill the measuring cup. Set aside.

Peel the grapefruit and divide into wedges. Cut each wedge in half and set aside.

Now, combine lemon,grapes, pineapple, and grapefruit in a juicer and process until juiced. Transfer to a serving glass and stir in the cinnamon.

Add some crushed ice and serve immediately.

Nutritional information per serving: Kcal: 230, Protein: 4g, Carbs: 69.1g, Fats: 1.1g

7.   Pepper Lettuce Juice

Ingredients:

1 large yellow bell pepper, chopped

1 cup of Romaine lettuce, chopped

1 cup of fennel, sliced

1 cup of cucumber, sliced

1 small zucchini, cubed

Preparation:

Wash the bell pepper and cut lengthwise in half. Remove the stem and seeds. Cut into small pieces and set aside.

Wash the Romaine lettuce thoroughly under cold running water. Drain and chop into small pieces. Set aside.

Trim off the fennel bulb and remove the green parts. Wash it and cut into small pieces. Fill the measuring cup and reserve the rest for later. Set aside.

Wash the cucumber and cut into thin slices. Fill the measuring cup and reserve the rest for later.

Wash the zucchini and cut into small cubes. Set aside.

Now, combine bell pepper, lettuce,fennel, cucumber, and zucchini in a juicer and process until juiced. Transfer to a serving glass and refrigerate for 5 minutes before serving.

Nutritional information per serving: Kcal: 85, Protein: 5.3g, Carbs: 25.2g, Fats: 1.1g

8. Cantaloupe Pear Juice

Ingredients:

1 cup of cantaloupe, peeled and chopped

1 medium-sized pear, chopped

1 whole leek, chopped

1 whole lime, peeled

1 oz of coconut water

¼ tsp of ginger, ground

Preparation:

Cut the cantaloupe in half. Scoop out the seeds and flesh. Cut and peel one large wedge. Chop into chunks and fill the measuring cup. Reserve the rest of the cantaloupe in a refrigerator.

Wash the pear lengthwise in half. Remove the core and cut into bite-sized pieces. Set aside.

Wash the leek thoroughly under cold running water. Drain and chop into small pieces. Set aside.

Peel the lime and cut lengthwise in half. Set aside.

Now, combine cantaloupe, pear, leek, and lime in a juicer and process until juiced. Transfer to a serving glass and stir in the coconut water and ginger.

Add some ice, or refrigerate for 5 minutes before serving.

Nutritional information per serving: Kcal: 184, Protein: 3.5g, Carbs: 56.2g, Fats: 0.8g

9.   Radish Brussels Sprout Juice

Ingredients:

2 large radishes, chopped

2 cups of Brussels sprouts, halved

1 small zucchini, chopped

1 cup of cucumber, sliced

2 large carrots, sliced

¼ tsp of turmeric, ground

Preparation:

Wash the radishes and trim off the green parts. Slightly peel and cut into small pieces. Set aside.

Wash the Brussels sprouts and trim off the outer layers. Cut into halves and fill the measuring cups. Reserve the rest in the refrigerator.

Wash the zucchini and cut into thin slices. Set aside.

Wash the cucumber and cut into thin slices. Fill the measuring cup and reserve the rest for later.

Wash and peel the carrots. Cut into thin slices and set aside.

Now, combine radishes, Brussels sprouts, zucchini, cucumber, and carrots in a juicer and process until juiced. Transfer to a serving glass and stir in the turmeric. Refrigerate for 15 minutes before serving.

Nutritional information per serving: Kcal: 118, Protein: 9.2g, Carbs: 35.7g, Fats: 1.3g

10.   Swiss Chard Lime Juice

Ingredients:

½ cup of Swiss chard

1 large lime, peeled

½ cup of fresh basil

2 large green apples, cored

¼ cup of fresh mint

Preparation:

Wash the Swiss chard and basil thoroughly and roughly chop it. Set aside.

Peel the lime and cut into quarters. Set aside.

Wash the mint leaves and soak in water for 10 minutes. Set aside.

Wash the apples and remove the core. Cut into bite-sized pieces and set aside.

Now combine, Swiss chard, lime, basil, and apples, and mint in a juicer. Process until juiced. Transfer to serving glasses and add some ice before serving.

Garnish with some extra mint leaves and add some ice before serving.

Enjoy!

Nutritional information per serving: Kcal: 114, Protein: 2.3g, Carbs: 30.4g, Fats: 0.2g

11.   Pomegranate Apple Juice

Ingredients:

½ cup of pomegranate seeds

1 large green apple, cored

½ cup of fresh kale

¼ tsp of ginger, ground

3-4 fresh mint leaves

Preparation:

Cut the top of the pomegranate fruit using a sharp knife. slice down to each of the white membranes inside of the fruit. Pop the seeds into a medium sized bowl.

Wash the apple and remove the core. Cut into bite-sized pieces and set aside.

Wash thoroughly the kale. Drain and roughly chop it. Set aside.

Process the pomegranate seeds, apple, and kale in a juicer until well juiced.

Transfer to serving glasses and stir in the ginger. Add some water to adjust the thickness and garnish with mint leaves.

Add few ice cubes and serve immediately.

Nutritional information per serving: Kcal: 143, Protein: 6.2g, Carbs: 41.2g, Fats: 2.4g

12.   Cucumber Pineapple Juice

Ingredients:

1 large cucumber

1 cup of pineapple, chopped

3 celery stalks

½ cup of fresh spinach

¼ tsp of ginger, ground

Preparation:

Wash and slice the cucumber into thick slices. Set aside.

Peel the pineapple and cut into chunks. Set aside.

Combine celery and spinach in a colander and wash under cold running water. Roughly chop the spinach and celery.

Combine cucumber, pineapple, celery, and spinach in a juicer and process until well juiced.

Transfer to serving glasses and stir in the ginger. Add a pinch of turmeric for some extra flavor. However, it's optional.

Serve immediately.

Nutritional information per serving: Kcal: 109, Protein: 3.3g, Carbs: 61.2g, Fats: 1.3g

13.   Broccoli Carrot Juice

Ingredients:

1 cup of fresh broccoli

4 large carrots

2 cups of cauliflower, chopped

1 large green apple, cored

1 small ginger root slice, 1-inch

Preparation:

Wash the broccoli and chop it into small pieces.

Wash the carrots and cut into small pieces.

Wash the apple and remove the core. Cut into bite-sized pieces and set aside.

Wash the cauliflower under cold running water, and place it in a medium-sized bowl. Chop into small pieces and add water enough to cover it. Set aside to soak for 15 minutes.

Peel the ginger root and cut into halves.

Now, process cauliflower, broccoli, apple, carrot, and ginger root. Transfer to serving glasses and add some ice cubes before serving.

Enjoy!

Nutritional information per serving: Kcal: 136, Protein: 6.3g, Carbs: 42.8g, Fats: 1.2g

14.   Sweet Potato Peach Juice

Ingredients:

2 medium-sized sweet potatoes, pre-cooked

1 large peach, pitted and halved

¼ tsp of ginger, ground

¼ tsp of cinnamon, ground

Preparation:

Peel the potatoes and place them in a pot of boiling water. Cook until fork-tender. Remove from the heat and drain well. Cut the potatoes into small pieces and set aside to cool completely.

Wash the peach and cut into halves. Remove the pit and chop into bite-sized pieces. Set aside.

Now, combine potatoes and peach in a juicer and process until juiced. Transfer to serving glasses and stir in the ginger and cinnamon.

Add some ice and serve immediately.

Nutritional information per serving: Kcal: 159, Protein: 5.2g, Carbs: 50.1g, Fats: 0.9g

15. Bok Choy Apple Juice

Ingredients:

1 small baby bok choy

1 large green apple, cored

¼ cup of fresh basil

1 medium-sized leek

2 large carrots

4-5 fresh kale leaves

Preparation:

Discard the ends of the bokchoy stems. Wash it thoroughly and chop it into small pieces. Set aside.

Wash the apple and remove the core. Cut into bite-sized pieces and set aside.

Wash the leek and chop into small pieces. set aside.

Combine basil and kale in a colander and wash under cold running water. Chop roughly with your hands. Set aside.

Wash the carrots and chop into thick slices. Set aside.

Now, process all prepared ingredients in a juicer. Transfer to serving glasses and refrigerate for 10 minutes before serving.

Enjoy!

Nutritional information per serving: Kcal: 169, Protein: 2.3g, Carbs: 46.2g, Fats: 1.9g

16.   Cantaloupe Lettuce Juice

Ingredients:

1 cup of cantaloupe, peeled

1 small Romaine lettuce head

1 tbsp of coconut, grated

½ cup of fresh basil

1 large cucumber

Preparation:

Peel the cantaloupe and cut into chunks. Reserve the rest of the cantaloupe in the refrigerator.

Wash the lettuce thoroughly. Roughly chop with hands and set aside.

Wash the cucumber and cut into thick slices. Set aside.

Wash the basil and chop with hands. Set aside.

Now, combine cantaloupe, lettuce, basil, and cucumber in a juicer and process until juiced.

Transfer to serving glasses and stir in the coconut. You can add some liquid honey for some extra taste, but this is optional.

Refrigerate for 15 minutes before serving.

Nutritional information per serving: Kcal: 112, Protein: 2.3g, Carbs: 22.6g, Fats: 1.1g

17. Mediterranean Citrus Juice

Ingredients:

½ tsp of fresh rosemary

3 large grapefruits, peeled

3 large oranges, peeled

1 whole lemon, peeled

Preparation:

Wash the grapefruits and cut into bite-sized pieces. Set aside.

Peel the oranges and divide into wedges. Set aside.

Peel the lemon and cut into quarters. Process in a juicer until well juiced.

Now, process grapefruits and oranges. Transfer to serving glasses and sprinkle with fresh rosemary for some extra flavor.

If you don't like rosemary, you can replace it with fresh mint.

Add some ice cubes and serve immediately.

Enjoy!

Nutritional information per serving: Kcal: 140, Protein: 3.4g, Carbs: 37.6g, Fats: 0.1g

18.   Orange Cucumber Juice

Ingredients:

2 large oranges, peeled

1 large cucumber, peeled

1 cup of broccoli

1 large carrot, sliced

Preparation:

Peel the oranges and cut into wedges.

Peel the cucumber and cut into bite-sized pieces and aside.

Wash the broccoli thoroughly. Cut into bite-sized pieces and set aside.

Wash and cut the carrot into thin slices. Process in a juicer until juiced. Now, continue to process broccoli, orange wedges, and cucumber.

Stir well with a spoon and add some ice cubes before serving.

Nutritional information per serving: Kcal: 68, Protein: 2.3g, Carbs: 19.7g, Fats: 0.1g

19. Fennel Pepper Juice

Ingredients:

1 large fennel bulb, trimmed

2 cups of fresh asparagus, trimmed

1 large green bell pepper, seeded

1 large yellow bell pepper, seeded

1 ginger root slice, 1-inch

2 oz of water

Preparation:

Wash the fennel bulb and trim off the wilted outer layers. Cut into small chunks and set aside.

Wash the bell peppers and cut in half. Remove the seeds and cut into small slices. Set aside.

Wash the asparagus and trim off the woody ends. Cut into 1-inch pieces and set aside.

Peel the ginger root slice and set aside.

Now, combine asparagus, fennel, green and yellow bell pepper, and ginger root in a juicer and process until juiced.

Transfer to serving glasses and stir in the water. Refrigerate for 5 minutes before serving and enjoy!

Nutrition information per serving: Kcal: 143, Protein: 12.1g, Carbs: 47.2g, Fats: 1.5g

20. Zucchini Lemon Juice

Ingredients:

1 large zucchini, chopped

1 large lemon, peeled

1 cup of pumpkin

1 medium-sized yellow apple, cored

1 medium-sized banana

2 oz of water

Preparation:

Peel the zucchini and cut in half. Scrape out the seeds with a spoon. Cut into chunks and set aside.

Peel the lemon and cut lengthwise in half. Set aside.

Peel the pumpkin and cut in half. Scoop out the seeds using a spoon. Cut one large wedge and peel it. Cut into small chunks and set aside. Reserve the rest for later.

Wash the apple and remove the core. Cut into bite-sized pieces and set aside.

Peel the banana and cut into small chunks. Set aside.

Now, process zucchini, lemon, pumpkin, apple, and banana in a juicer. Transfer to serving glasses and stir in the water.

Add some ice and serve immediately.

Nutrition information per serving: Kcal: 254, Protein: 7.5g, Carbs: 72.9g, Fats: 1.9g

21.   Green Celery Juice

Ingredients:

1 cup of celery

1 cup of Swiss chards

1 medium-sized apple, cored

1 cup of collard greens

2 tbsp of fresh parsley

4-5 fresh spinach leaves

2 oz of water

Preparation:

Combine Swiss chards, collard greens, celery, and spinach in a colander. Wash thoroughly under cold running water and drain. Torn with hands and set aside.

Wash the apple and remove the core. Cut into bite-sized pieces and set aside.

Now, combine Swiss chards, celery, apple, collard greens, and spinach in a juicer and process until juiced.

Transfer to serving glasses and stir in the water. Add some ice and garnish with fresh parsley.

Enjoy!

Nutrition information per serving: Kcal: 106, Protein: 4.8g, Carbs: 31.3g, Fats: 1.1g

22.   Broccoli Artichoke Juice

Ingredients:

1 cup of fresh broccoli

1 large artichoke head

1 cup of Brussels sprouts, trimmed

1 large lemon, peeled

1 large cucumber

3 tbsp of fresh parsley

Preparation:

Wash the broccoli and chop into small pieces. set aside.

Using a sharp knife, trim off the outer layers of the artichoke. Wash it and cut into bite-sized pieces. Set aside.

Wash the Brussels sprouts and trim off the outer layers. Cut in half and set aside.

Peel the lemon and cut lengthwise in half. Set aside.

Wash the cucumber and cut into thick slices. Set aside.

Now, process Brussels sprouts, broccoli, artichoke, lemon, and cucumber in a juicer.

Transfer to serving glasses and garnish with fresh parsley. Refrigerate for 10 minutes before serving.

Enjoy!

Nutrition information per serving: Kcal: 140, Protein: 13.8g, Carbs: 48.1g, Fats: 1.4g

23. Apple Lemon Juice

Ingredients:

2 medium-sized Golden Delicious apples

1 large lemon, peeled

1 large cucumber

3 medium-sized celery stalks

A handful of spinach

2 oz of water

Preparation:

Wash the apples and remove the core. Cut into bite-sized pieces and set aside.

Peel the lemon and cut lengthwise in half. Set aside.

Wash the cucumber and cut into thick slices. Set aside.

Wash the celery stalks and cut into 1-inch pieces. Set aside.

Wash the spinach thoroughly and torn with hands. Set aside.

Now, process apples, lemon, cucumber, celery, and spinach in a juicer. Transfer to serving glasses and stir in the water.

Add some ice and serve.

Nutrition information per serving: Kcal: 224, Protein: 5.2g, Carbs: 65.4g, Fats: 1.5g

24.   Swiss Chard Cucumber Juice

Ingredients:

2 cups of Swiss chard

1 large cucumber

1 cup of fresh parsley, torn

1 small yellow apple, cored

1 small orange, peeled

Preparation:

Combine parsley and Swiss chard in a colander and wash thoroughly under cold running water. Drain and torn with hands. Set aside.

Wash the cucumber and cut into thick slices. Set aside.

Wash the apple and remove the core. Cut into bite-sized pieces and set aside.

Peel the orange and divide into wedges. Set aside.

Now, combine parsley, Swiss chard, cucumber apple, and orange in a juicer and process until juiced. Transfer to serving glasses and add some ice before serving.

Enjoy!

Nutrition information per serving: Kcal: 161, Protein: 6.3g, Carbs: 46.3g, Fats: 1.2g

25. Mint Arugula Juice

Ingredients:

1 cup of fresh mint

1 cup of fresh arugula

1 large carrot

1 large orange, peeled

1 large red bell pepper, seeded

Preparation:

Combine mint and arugula in a colander and wash thoroughly under cold running water. Drain and torn with hands. Set aside.

Wash the carrot and cut into thick slices. Set aside.

Peel the orange and divide into wedges. Set aside.

Wash the bell pepper and cut in half. Remove the seeds and chop into small slices. Set aside.

Now, combine mint, arugula, carrot, orange, and bell pepper in a juicer and process until juiced.

Transfer to serving glasses and stir in the water. You can add a pinch of Himalayan salt, but this is optional.

Add some ice and serve immediately.

Nutrition information per serving: Kcal: 153, Protein: 7.9g, Carbs: 47.3g, Fats: 1.3g

26.   Plum Ginger Juice

Ingredients:

5 large plums, pitted

1 cup of fresh broccoli

1 large cucumber

1 medium-sized apple, cored

¼ tsp of ginger, ground

Preparation:

Wash the plums and cut in half. Remove the pits and set aside.

Wash the broccoli and cut into small pieces. Set aside.

Wash the cucumber and cut into thick slices and set aside.

Wash the apple and remove the core. Cut into bite-sized pieces and set aside.

Now, combine plums, broccoli, cucumber, and apple in a juicer and process until juiced.

Transfer to serving glasses and stir in the ginger. Add few ice cubes before serving.

Enjoy!

Nutrition information per serving: Kcal: 268, Protein: 7.6g, Carbs: 77.4g, Fats: 1.9g

27. Pomegranate Lime Juice

Ingredients:

1 cup of pomegranate seeds

1 large lime, peeled

1 cup of beets, trimmed and chopped

2 large carrots

1 large cucumber

Preparation:

Cut the top of the pomegranate fruit using a sharp knife. Slice down to each of the white membranes inside of the fruit. Pop the seeds into a measuring cup and set aside.

Peel the lime and cut into lengthwise in half. Set aside.

Wash the beets and trim off the green parts. Cut into bite-sized pieces and fill the measuring cup. Reserve the rest for some other juice.

Wash the carrot and cucumber and cut into thick slices. Set aside.

Now, process pomegranate seeds, lime, beets, carrots and cucumber in a juicer.

Transfer to serving glasses and stir in the water. Add some ice and serve!

Nutrition information per serving: Kcal: 194, Protein: 7.2g, Carbs: 57.7g, Fats: 1.9g

28.   Beet Cauliflower Juice

Ingredients:

3 large beets, trimmed

1 cup of cauliflower, chopped

2 cups of green grapes

1 large lemon, peeled

Preparation:

Wash the beets and trim off the green parts. Cut into bite-sized pieces and set

aside.

Trim off the outer leaves of cauliflower. Wash it and cut into small pieces. Fill the measuring cup and reserve the rest for some other juice. Set aside.

Wash the green grapes under cold running water. Set aside.

Peel the lemon and cut lengthwise in half. Set aside.

Now, process beets, grapes, cauliflower, and lemon in a juicer.

Transfer to serving glasses and add some ice cubes before serving.

Enjoy!

Nutrition information per serving: Kcal: 226, Protein: 7.8g, Carbs: 65.8g, Fats: 1.5g

29.   Orange Carrot Juice

Ingredients:

4 large oranges, peeled

1 cup of carrots, sliced

1 cup of broccoli, chopped

1 cup of Brussels sprouts, chopped

1 cup of turnip greens, chopped

1 tbsp of honey

¼ cup of pure coconut water

Preparation:

Peel the oranges and divide into wedges. Set aside.

Wash the carrots and cut into thick slices. Set aside.

Wash the broccoli and cut into small pieces. Set aside.

Wash the Brussels sprouts and trim off the outer layers. Cut in half and set aside.

Wash the turnip greens thoroughly and torn with hands. Set aside.

Now, combine broccoli, Brussels sprouts, carrots, turnip greens, and oranges in a juicer and process until juiced.

Transfer to serving glasses and stir in the honey and coconut water. Add some ice cubes before serving or refrigerate for 5 minutes.

Enjoy!

Nutrition information per serving: Kcal: 367, Protein: 14.47g, Carbs: 116g, Fats: 1.9g

30.   Blackberry Orange Juice

Ingredients:

1 cup of blackberries, fresh

1 large orange, peeled

2 wedges of watermelon, seeded

½ cup of pure coconut water, unsweetened

1 tbsp of honey, raw

Preparation:

Wash the blackberries under cold running water and set aside.

Peel the orange and divide into wedges. Set aside.

Cut the watermelon lengthwise. Cut two large wedges and peel them. Cut into chunks and remove the seeds. Set aside.

Now, combine watermelon, blackberries, and orange in a juicer and process until juiced.

Transfer to serving glasses and stir the coconut water and honey.

Refrigerate for 5 minutes before serving.

Enjoy!

Nutrition information per serving: Kcal: 264, Protein: 7.2g, Carbs: 78.6g, Fats: 1.7g

31. Tomato Pepper Juice

Ingredients:

2 large tomatoes, peeled

1 cup of red bell peppers, chopped and seeds removed

4 cups of watercress, torn

4 cups of red leaf lettuce, torn

¼ cup of water

Preparation:

Wash the tomatoes and place them in a bowl. Cut into quarters and reserve the juice while cutting. Set aside.

Wash the bell peppers and cut in half. Remove the seeds and roughly chop it. Fill the measuring cup and reserve the rest for some other juice. Set aside.

Combine watercress and red leaf lettuce in a colander. Wash thoroughly under cold running water and torn with hands. Set aside.

Now, combine tomatoes, bell pepper, watercress, and red leaf lettuce in a juicer and process until juiced.

Transfer to serving glasses and stir in the reserved tomato juice and water.

Refrigerate for 5 minutes before serving.

Enjoy!

Nutrition information per serving: Kcal: 106, Protein: 9.2g, Carbs: 27.4g, Fats: 1.5g

32.   Lemon Zucchini Juice

Ingredients:

1 whole lemon, peeled and halved

1 small zucchini, thinly sliced

1 cup of cauliflower, chopped

1 medium artichoke, chopped

1 small ginger knob, chopped

¼ tsp salt

Preparation:

Peel the lemon and cut lengthwise in half. Set aside.

Wash the zucchini and thinly slice it. Set aside.

Trim off the outer layer of the cauliflower. Cut into bite-sized pieces and wash it. Fill the measuring cup and sprinkle with some salt. Set aside.

Trim off the outer layers of the artichoke using a sharp paring knife. Cut into bite-sized pieces and set aside.

Peel the ginger knob and chop into small pieces. Set aside.

Now, combine lemon, zucchini, cauliflower, artichoke, and

ginger in a juicer. Process until well juiced.

Transfer to a serving glass and refrigerate for 10 minutes before serving.

Enjoy!

Nutrition information per serving: Kcal: 82, Protein: 8.4g, Carbs: 28.9g, Fats: 1.1g

33.   Broccoli Parsley Juice

Ingredients:

2 cups of broccoli, chopped

1 cup of fresh parsley, torn

1 cup of beets, trimmed and chopped

1 cup of celery, chopped

¼ tsp of turmeric, ground

¼ tsp ginger, ground

Preparation:

Wash the broccoli and trim off the outer layers. Chop into small pieces and set aside.

Rinse the parsley under cold running water and slightly drain. Torn with hands into small pieces and set aside.

Wash and peel the beets. Trim off the green ends and chop into bite-sized pieces. Fill the measuring cup and reserve the rest for later.

Wash the celery stalks and chop it into bite-sized pieces. Fill the measuring cup and set aside.

Now, combine broccoli, parsley, beets, and celery in a juicer and process until juiced. Transfer to a serving glass and stir in the turmeric and ginger.

Refrigerate for 5 minutes before serving.

Nutrition information per serving: Kcal: 109, Protein: 9.8g, Carbs: 31.8g, Fats: 1.5g

34.   Banana Blackberry Juice

Ingredients:

1 cup of blackberries

1 large banana, chunked

1 cup of mango, chunked

1 large orange, peeled

¼ tsp of cinnamon, ground

Preparation:

Place the blackberries in a colander and wash under cold running water. Slightly drain and set aside.

Peel the banana and cut into small chunks. Set aside.

Wash the mango and cut into small chunks. Fill the measuring cup and reserve the rest for later.

Peel the orange and divide into wedges. Cut each wedge in half and set aside.

Now, combine mango, blackberries, banana, and orange in a juicer and process until juiced. Transfer to a serving glass and stir in the cinnamon.

Add few ice cubes and serve immediately.

Nutrition information per serving: Kcal: 296, Protein: 6.6g, Carbs: 91.2g, Fats: 2.1g

35.   Lime Blueberry Juice

Ingredients:

1 whole lime, peeled

1 cup of blueberries

1 cup of fresh spinach, chopped

1 medium-sized orange

1 oz coconut water

1 tbsp fresh mint, torn

Preparation:

Peel the lime and cut lengthwise in half. Set aside.

Place the blueberries in a colander and wash under cold running water. Slightly drain and set aside.

Wash the spinach thoroughly and drain. Chop into small pieces and set aside.

Peel the orange and divide into wedges. Cut each wedge in half and set aside.

Now, combine blueberries, spinach, lime, and orange in a juicer and process until well juiced. Transfer to a serving glass and stir in the coconut water.

Sprinkle with some fresh mint and serve.

Enjoy!

Nutrition information per serving: Kcal: 158, Protein: 8.5g, Carbs: 48.1g, Fats: 1.5g

36.   Tomato Basil Juice

Ingredients:

1 cup of cherry tomatoes, halved

1 cup of Swiss chard, torn

1 cup of basil, torn

1 cup of beets, trimmed

¼ tsp of balsamic vinegar

¼ tsp of salt

1 oz of water

Preparation:

Wash the cherry tomatoes and remove the green stems. Cut in half and fill the measuring cup. Reserve the rest in the refrigerator for some other juice.

Combine basil and Swiss chard in a large colander and rinse thoroughly under cold running water. Drain and torn with hands into small pieces. Set aside.

Wash the beets and trim off the green parts. Cut into thin slices and fill the measuring cup. Reserve the rest for later.

Now, combine cherry tomatoes, Swiss chard, basil, and beets in a juicer and process until juiced. Transfer to a serving glass and stir in the vinegar, salt, and water.

Serve immediately.

Nutrition information per serving: Kcal: 72, Protein: 5.1g, Carbs: 21.6g, Fats: 0.7g

37. Orange Pear Juice

Ingredients:

1 medium-sized orange, peeled

1 medium-sized pear, chopped

1 cup of fennel, chopped

1 whole lemon, peeled

¼ tsp of cinnamon, ground

1 oz of coconut water

Preparation:

Peel the orange and divide into wedges. Cut each wedge in half and set aside.

Wash the pear and cut in half. Remove the core and cut into small pieces. Set aside.

Trim off the outer wilted layers of the fennel. Roughly chop it and fill the measuring cup. Reserve the rest for later.

Peel the lemon and cut lengthwise in half. Set aside.

Now, combine orange, pear, fennel, and lemon in a juicer and process until well juiced. Transfer to a serving glass and stir in the cinnamon and coconut water.

Refrigerate for 10 minutes before serving.

Enjoy!

Nutrition information per serving: Kcal: 156, Protein: 3.6g, Carbs: 54.2g, Fats: 0.7g

38. Carrot Lemon Juice

Ingredients:

1 large carrot, sliced

1 whole lemon, peeled

1 cup of celery, chopped

1 small Granny Smith's apple, cored

¼ tsp ginger, ground

Preparation:

Wash and peel the carrot. Cut into small slices and set aside.

Wash the celery and cut into small pieces. Set aside.

Peel the lemon and cut lengthwise in half. Set aside.

Wash the apple and cut in half. Remove the core and cut into bite-sized pieces. Set aside.

Now, combine carrot, celery, lemon, and apple in a juicer and process until juiced. Transfer to a serving glass and stir in the water and ginger. Refrigerate for 5 minutes.

Serve immediately.

Nutrition information per serving: Kcal: 105, Protein: 2.4g, Carbs: 32.8g, Fats: 0.7g

39. Pear Cucumber Juice

Ingredients:

1 large pear, chopped

1 whole cucumber, sliced

1 cup of purple cabbage, chopped

1 whole lemon, peeled

Preparation:

Wash the pear and cut lengthwise in half. Remove the core and chop into small pieces. Set aside.

Wash the cucumber and cut into thin slices. Set aside.

Wash the cabbage thoroughly under cold running water. Drain and chop into small pieces. Set aside.

Peel the lemon and cut lengthwise in half. Set aside.

Now, combine pear, cucumber, cabbage, and lemon in a juicer. Process until well juiced. Transfer to a serving glass and serve immediately.

Enjoy!

Nutrition information per serving: Kcal: 173, Protein: 4.7g, Carbs: 57.9g, Fats: 0.9g

40. Kale Pomegranate Juice

Ingredients:

1 cup of fresh kale, torn

1 cup of pomegranate seeds

2 cups of Swiss chard, torn

1 large orange, peeled

1 small Golden Delicious apple, cored

Preparation:

Cut the top of the pomegranate fruit using a sharp paring knife. Slice down to each of the white membranes inside of the fruit. Pop the seeds into a measuring cup and set aside.

Combine Swiss chard and kale in a large colander. Rinse under cold running water and drain. Torn into small pieces and set aside.

Peel the orange and divide into wedges. Cut each wedge in half and set aside.

Wash the apple and cut lengthwise in half. Remove the core and cut into bite-sized pieces. Set aside.

Now, combine Swiss chard, kale, pomegranate seeds, orange, and apple in a juicer and process until juiced. Transfer to a serving glass and add few ice cubes.

Serve immediately.

Nutrition information per serving: Kcal: 227, Protein: 7.9g, Carbs: 66.1g, Fats: 2.3g

41.   Salted Avocado Zucchini Juice

Ingredients:

1 cup of avocado, cubed

1 small zucchini, sliced

3 large radishes, chopped

1 cup of celery, chopped

1 cup of cucumber, sliced

¼ tsp of salt

1 oz of water

Preparation:

Peel the avocado and cut in half. Remove the pit and cut into small cubes. Fill the measuring cup and reserve the rest for later.

Wash the zucchini and cut into thin slices. Set aside.

Wash the radishes and cut into small pieces. Set aside.

Wash the celery and chop it into bite-sized pieces. Set aside.

Wash the cucumber and cut into thin slices. Fill the

measuring cup and reserve the rest for later. Set aside.

Now, combine avocado, radishes, zucchini, celery, and cucumber in a juicer and process until juiced. Transfer to a serving glass and stir in the salt and water.

Serve immediately.

Nutrition information per serving: Kcal: 235, Protein: 5.6g, Carbs: 22.3g, Fats: 22.6g

42. Artichoke Lime Juice

Ingredients:

1 medium-sized artichoke, chopped

1 whole lime, peeled

1 cup of basil, torn

1 cup of cucumber, sliced

2 oz of water

Preparation:

Trim off the outer leaves of the artichoke. Wash it and chop into small pieces. Set aside.

Peel the lime and cut lengthwise in half. Set aside.

Wash the basil thoroughly under cold running water. Drain and torn into small pieces. Set aside.

Wash the cucumber and cut into thin slices. Fill the measuring cup and reserve the rest in the refrigerator.

Now, combine artichoke, lime, basil, and cucumber in a juicer and process until juiced. Transfer to a serving glass and stir in the water.

Refrigerate for 5 minutes before serving.

Nutrition information per serving: Kcal: 53, Protein: 5.5g, Carbs: 19.6g, Fats: 0.4g

43.   Tomato Collard Green Juice

Ingredients:

1 large tomato

1 cup of collard greens, torn

2 cups of parsnips, trimmed

1 large yellow bell pepper, seeded

1 large cucumber

Preparation:

Wash the tomato and place in a bowl. Cut into quarters and reserve the juice while cutting. Set aside.

Wash the collard greens thoroughly and torn with hands. Set aside.

Wash the parsnips and cut into thick slices. Set aside.

Wash the bell pepper and cut in half. Remove the seeds and cut into small pieces. Set aside.

Wash the cucumber and cut into thick slices. Set aside.

Now, process parsnips, bell pepper, tomato, collard greens, and cucumber in a juicer.

Transfer to serving glasses and stir in the reserved tomato juice.

Refrigerate for 10 minutes before serving.

Nutritional information per serving: Kcal: 254, Protein: 9.5g, Carbs: 77.7g, Fats: 2.2g

44. Spinach Cilantro Juice

Ingredients:

½ cup of fresh spinach

½ cup of fresh cilantro

½ cup of fresh arugula

3-4 celery stalks

1 large green apple, cored

Preparation:

Combine spinach, cilantro, and arugula in a large colander. Wash under cold running water and drain. Torn into small pieces and set aside.

Wash the celery stalks and cut into small pieces. Set aside.

Wash the apple and remove the core. Cut into bite-sized pieces and set aside.

Now, combine arugula, cilantro, spinach, celery, and apple in a juicer and process until juiced.

Transfer to serving glasses and add few ice cubes before serving.

Enjoy!

Nutritional information per serving: Kcal: 61, Protein: 2.1g, Carbs: 20.2g, Fats: 1.2g

45.   Cherry Lemon Juice

Ingredients:

1 cup of fresh cherries, pitted

1 large lemon, peeled

1 cup of mango, cubed

1 cup of watermelon, cubed

1 tbsp of liquid honey

2 oz of water

Preparation:

Wash the cherries under cold running water. Drain and cut in half. Remove the pits and set aside.

Peel the lemon and cut lengthwise in half. Set aside.

Peel the mango and cut into small chunks. Set aside.

Cut the watermelon lengthwise. For one cup, you will need about 1 large wedge. Peel and cut into chunks. Remove the seeds and set aside. Reserve the rest of the melon for some other juices.

Now, process cherries, mango, lemon, and watermelon in a juicer.

Transfer to serving glasses and add few ice cubes before serving.

Enjoy!

Nutrition information per serving: Kcal: 288, Protein: 4.6g, Carbs: 68.3g, Fats: 1.3g

46.   Orange Squash Juice

Ingredients:

1 large orange, peeled

1 cup of butternut squash, cubed

1 cup of avocado, peeled, pitted, and cubed

1 cup of fresh basil

1 large lime, peeled

2 oz of coconut water

Preparation:

Peel the orange and divide into wedges. Set aside.

Peel the butternut squash and remove the seeds using a spoon. Cut into small cubes and reserve the rest of the squash for some other recipe. Wrap in a plastic foil and refrigerate.

Peel the avocado in half. Remove the pit and cut into small chunks. Set aside.

Wash the basil thoroughly and torn with hands. Set aside.

Peel the lime and cut lengthwise in half. Set aside.

Now, process avocado, squash, basil, orange, and lime in a juicer.

Transfer to serving glasses and add few ice cubes before serving.

Nutrition information per serving: Kcal: 339, Protein: 6.9g, Carbs: 56.7g, Fats: 21.9g

47.   Cayenne Leek Juice

Ingredients:

2 large leeks

1 cup of asparagus, trimmed

1 large artichoke head

1 garlic clove, peeled

1 large cucumber

¼ tsp of Cayenne pepper

¼ tsp of Himalayan salt

Preparation:

Wash the leeks and chop into small pieces. Set aside.

Wash the asparagus and trim off the woody ends. Cut into small pieces and set aside.

Trim off the outer leaves of the artichoke using a sharp knife. Wash it and cut into small pieces. Set aside.

Peel the garlic clove and set aside.

Wash the cucumber and cut into thick slices. Set aside.

Now, process asparagus, leeks, artichoke, garlic, and cucumber in a juicer.

Transfer to serving glasses and stir in the Himalayan salt and Cayenne pepper.

Refrigerate for 30 minutes before serving.

Nutrition information per serving: Kcal: 245, Protein: 14.2g, Carbs: 71.9g, Fats: 1.5g

ADDITIONAL TITLES FROM THIS AUTHOR

70 Effective Meal Recipes to Prevent and Solve Being Overweight: Burn Fat Fast by Using Proper Dieting and Smart Nutrition

By Joe Correa CSN

48 Acne Solving Meal Recipes: The Fast and Natural Path to Fixing Your Acne Problems in Less Than 10 Days!

By Joe Correa CSN

41 Alzheimer's Preventing Meal Recipes: Reduce or Eliminate Your Alzheimer's Condition in 30 Days or Less!

By Joe Correa CSN

70 Effective Breast Cancer Meal Recipes: Prevent and Fight Breast Cancer with Smart Nutrition and Powerful Foods

By Joe Correa CSN